Praise for
looking into your voice
the poetic and eccentric realities of alzheimer's

The questions posed by this book are brilliant—they are questions that many people would never think to ask anyone else, let alone someone with Alzheimer's, but they are the ones that are most important. Not only care-partners and Alzheimer's organizations, but also society at large, are well served by the insight contained here.
LYNN JACKSON *Diagnosed with early stage dementia; co-founder, Dementia Advocacy and Support Network International (DASNI)*

Brave, playful, and inspiring—this little book manages to capture the enormity of all that is Alzheimer's with elegant simplicity.
ANNE DAVIS BASTING *Ph.D., Director of the UWM Center on Age & Community and author of* Forget Memory: Creating Better Lives for People with Dementia

Tender and stark, these poetic dialogues between a mother and daughter provide a moving glimpse into both the losses suffered and insights gained when living with Alzheimer's disease.
KELLY DUFFIN *CEO, Alzheimer Society of Canada*

Heartbreaking and beautiful . . . Cathie Borrie has discovered the poetry in her mother's musings. Unfettered as a result of Alzheimer's disease, they fly freely, communicating both a fresh appreciation of the infinite possibilities of words and her mother's enduring, essential humanity.
MARY S. MITTELMAN *DrPH, Director, Psychosocial Research and Support, Center of Excellence on Brain Aging; co-author,* Counseling the Alzheimer's Caregiver: A Resource for Healthcare Professionals

This book is living proof of the inventiveness and profundity of one individual with dementia. It is a little gem of little gems, and a triumph of creativity over adversity. Out of memory loss comes the unforgettable.
JOHN KILLICK *Poet; Writer-in-Residence at the Dementia Services Development Centre, University of Stirling*

A kaleidoscope of the tangled web of human relationships that illuminates the human capacity for love, the recall of precious moments and the shifting sands of the Alzheimer's mind.
GLEN REES CEO, *Alzheimer's Australia*

In the mesmerizing currents of this important work, a searching but sure voice delivers us from rational ideas into the magic of a new kind of language. If we let ourselves look into this voice and hear its music, we can move into the embrace of poetry and the sacred space of love.
ELLEN S. JAFFE *M.A., Poet; teacher; psychotherapist*

I read Cathie Borrie's beautiful and poetic book with tears in my eyes and a smile on my face. Her conversations with her mother show us how much we can still learn from minds that are tangled with plaques. How fortunate we are that Cathie has shared with us these original, fresh, and poignant communications between two loving, humorous, and wise people. *looking into your voice ~ the poetic and eccentric realities of alzheimer's* is a gift you should give yourself and others.
JUDITH FOX *Author of* I Still Do: Loving and Living with Alzheimer's

In this tender and moving collection, brief snatches of conversation throw out haunting observations from, and startling insights into, a mind we might wrongly think incapable. There is sometimes impeccable logic in them, more often a slightly offkey note akin to poetry. It is a beautiful testimony to the resilience of the human spirit, well worth meditating upon.
JOAN COLDWELL *Publisher, Hedgerow Press*

In the "upside-down language of birds" Borrie and her mother find each other. This book challenges our beliefs about what it means to live with dementia and strengthens our knowledge of the possibilities of the mind. More, it's a belly laugh—and that is smart medicine.
GARY GLAZNER *Founder and Executive Director of the Alzheimer's Poetry Project*

Une explosion et l'Ésprit s'ouvre, se dilate . . . This book shows us that dementia—a term to describe our incapacity to understand and celebrate the metamorphosis of a mind—can be a way to access and experience the extreme richness and flourishing of the human psyche. *looking into your voice ~ the poetic and eccentric realities of alzheimer's* is a work of art that captures the work of art of an altering reality. An illumination of the strange and beautiful symphonic shifting of the dementia mind, it brings forth startling and visionary truth.
DARIO GARAU SETZU *Pianist; musicologist; researcher; visionary caregiver*

It's a good thing when the veil lifts as it does in this work. What previously felt opaque suddenly offers a view of life that shines. This book reminds me that when I listen in a new way, a window to the soul is eased open. That's a relief . . . and it's also redemptive.
JOHN FOX *President, CEO, The Institute for Poetic Medicine; author of* Poetic Medicine: The Healing Art of Poem-Making

looking into your voice
the poetic and eccentric realities of alzheimer's

A collection of recorded conversations between
Cathie Borrie & her mother, Joan Borrie

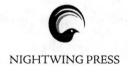

NIGHTWING PRESS

Library and Archives Canada Cataloguing in Publication

Borrie, Cathie
Looking into your voice : the poetic and eccentric realities
of Alzheimer's / Cathie Borrie.

Quotations spoken by Joan Borrie, also published in The long hello.
ISBN 978-0-9813786-7-1

1. Borrie, Joan--Quotations. 2. Alzheimer's disease--Patients--
Language. 3. Alzheimer's disease--Patients--Care--British Columbia--
Vancouver. I. Borrie, Joan II. Title.

RC523.B674 2010   616.8'31   C2010-904527-0

Cover art: Dean Goelz, NYC
Cover design Jonathan Wolferstan
Book design: J.L. Saloff
Author photo: Kimberly Mara, Eclipse Photography
Photo of Cathie and Joan Borrie: Sarah Solano
NIGHTWING PRESS logo: Tom Graney

Printed on acid-free paper.

NIGHTWING PRESS

ALSO BY CATHIE BORRIE

The Long Hello ~ The Other Side of Alzheimer's
(paperback, ebook and audiobook)

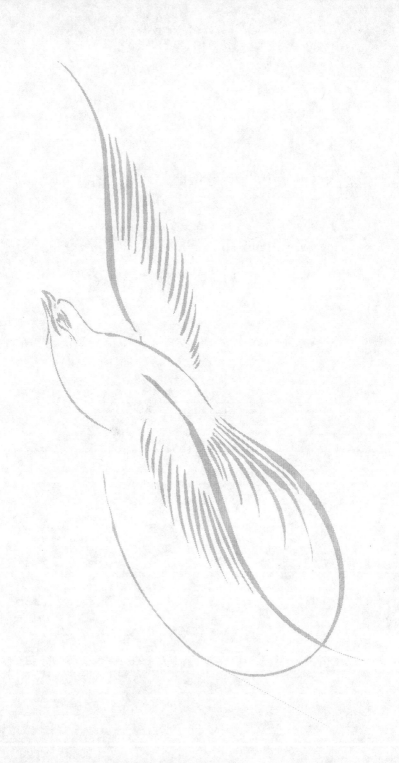

I felt free,
free and undivided,
free as a bird...

Are you sure I'm eighty-six?

         Yes, how old did you think you were?

I didn't know whether I was going that way
or that way.

         What did you think you were doing?

               I thought I was going

    in-between.

All I know is

I've been zapped of my strength.

Yes,

and all the funny little laughs.

I've been zapped of them all.

Zapped.

Did you have anywhere to go with my mind?

No, I thought I would leave it right
where it is. That's safer, no?

But where did you put all that information?

In my head.

Oh dear.

It doesn't matter, does it?

Not unless a car is coming!

Listen, a bird!

What are the birds saying?

They're chirping.

In a language?

In their language.

In an upside-down language.

What do you think about the sky?

Oh I don't know about the sky
I don't really know about it.

It's pretty beautiful
but you have to wear gloves because it puts
fingerprints on it

and you don't want that.

I've reached the ultimate of the intimate
and that's the end of it.

If I'm not here it's not my house.

How are you?

You mean, eventually?

_Well, happy 8 out of 10. You see,
it's my root section and I can't let it down._

Even if it lets me down.

Time is running out. That awful feeling of
time
running out
is now backed up.

Well, maybe someone will turn the clock around.

I love listening to you talk.

You love what?

Listening to you talk.

Oh. I thought I heard you say, 'I love looking into your voice.'

I love that
too.

I think I'm more concentrated,
and, sort of.

I sort of, am.

It's become part of me.

Something has gone, something bad has gone.

I think we reached the limit of our soul of misery and we're now   poof

and we're just doing the best we can.

We're not feeling like that

       we just do

       we just are.

I think that's the way it is.

I am writing down a lot of things you say.

Don't think for a moment it's foolproof.

Do you know who I am?

Do you?

What do you think
is the nicest thing about you?

Nothing.

Okay.
What's the second nicest thing?

My love of music,
my love of good music.

In fact, it might be the first thing.

You're getting pretty funny.

Do you mean funny, queer?

I mean funny, amusing.
It's a fine line though, isn't it?

It is with me.

I haven't any tears if that's what you're wondering.

Do you think when we die
we'll see people we know?

*I don't know, and I don't know
anyone who would.*

What's so scary about dying?

Well, have you ever tried it?

What happens after we die?

I don't know, I was never there.

What happens to animals when they die?

They go back to their roots.

How do they find their way back?

In their organs.
        They sniff and smell their way back.

Look,

                          the trees outside your window are so
                                                lush!

Yes love, lush, and the fish jumping out of
the sea.

You are like the sea . . .
tide going in, tide going out

storms

beautiful sky

                                          full of fish.

Is your hand bothering you?

No, it's much better than last night. Last night, this finger here was giving all the answers.

What's the worst thing a person could do to
another person?

*They could throw their sublime
into the ridiculous.*

I feel rather soured by everyone and everything, and am not amused by a kettle of fish.

You're feeling better today, aren't you?

Yes.

Because?

Because it's all coming in and none going out.

How would you like us to be related?

I think we're doing fine in the water.

Which do you like better,
the moon or the stars?

The moon.

Because?

It's more beautiful.

In what way?

It's more lonely, isn't it?

That girl,
she was the one I found most fascinating, but I always
thought she employed far too much use of the wind.

What does sorrow mean?

It's a form of sadness, brought about
on a gray and heavy day.

I just stamp my foot and there she isn't.

I felt free, free and undivided, free as a bird!
That I don't owe anyone anything.

I feel refreshed.

Free to flap my arms like a bird.

Go where I want to go.

Do what I want to do.

This business has been on and off, on and off. If they'd just put their foot to the floor, we'd know

                                         where we are.

I just wish someone would let the old people know

                                         what's going on.

I jump up

            like a startled gazelle,

                          and then

the prayer comes around.

I want to cut some of the brambles down, some of the old stuff. And it's all different, but that's what I'm signing for.

I dreamt last night that I had come back here, back from being up in the valley of a thousand deaths.

Why do people marry?

For two reasons.

They want to fill up their boots, and they want to keep going, and they don't care where.

*When did the sheets for sarcasm come
around?*

What is love?

It's the sublime felt between two people

in the same working order.

Cathie was up here and she said to me,

'Mum, I'm not going to offer to

give them my shadow.'

Where was this?

Somewhere on the other side

of here.

All the sides
were lit up
and not convergent.

I don't think there's anything more we can say

*because everything we want to know is really on there
. . . who is in charge and what they're doing and all
the rest*

*And so I think that that's about it. It sort of ends the
story right now,   for now.*

Will there be more stories?

Oh yes, a lot more.

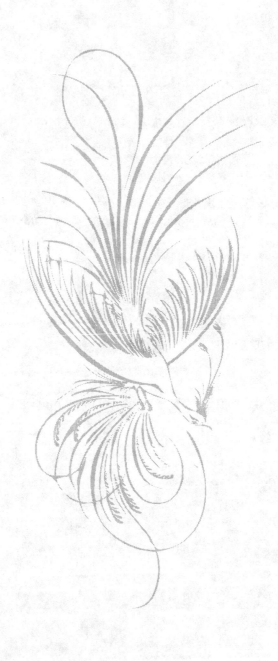

GRATITUDE

Special thanks for rendering my mother's words in poetic form must go to Dianna Hurford, whose tongue is crowned with laurels.

Dianna Hurford is a creative consultant and poet. She co-authored (with Wendy Sarkissian) the book *Creative Community Planning: Transformative Engagement Methods of Working at the Edge* (2010).

POSTSCRIPT

looking into your voice ~ the poetic and eccentric realities of alzheimer's

is a collection of conversations offering alternative and beautiful insights into the Alzheimer's mind. These vignettes are from Cathie Borrie's lyrical memoir, *The Long Hello ~ The Other Side of Alzheimer's*, which chronicles and cherishes the relationship between a mother and daughter over a seven-year period as the mother's mind transforms and her dementia increases. The mother's voice weaves throughout the memoir with insight, humor and an astonishing poetic sensibility, challenging the negative stereotypes pervasive in the current and often limiting geography of dementia.

BOOKS, READINGS, AND SPEAKING ENGAGEMENTS

Mailing list, blog, purchasing information, other books and editions, updates:

Website: www.cathieborrie.com
Email: cathieborrie@gmail.com
       cb@cathieborrie.com

Facebook: Cathie Borrie
Twitter: @cathieborrie
Linkedin: @Cathie Borrie

Cathie Borrie's memoir *The Long Hello ~ The Other Side of Alzheimer's* is available in paperback, ebook, and audiobook (read by writer and actor Melia McClure)

AUTHOR BIO

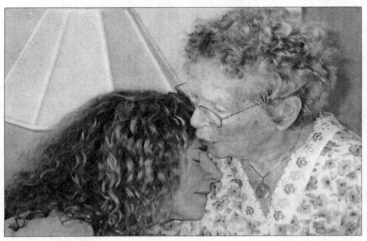

Sarah Solano

Cathie Borrie (a.k.a. Cath, CB, Cat) has degrees in health (2) and law (1), but nothing prepared her for the seven years she spent caring for her mother who had Alzheimer's and Parkinson's. Along this heartbreaking and unexpectedly fascinating journey, she discovered that recording conversations with her mother, writing a memoir, and learning to ballroom dance were ways to tell both her and her mother's stories.

Excerpts from her memoir *The Long Hello* were shortlisted three times in the CBC (Canadian Broadcasting Corporation) Literary Awards, Canada's most notable writing competition for unpublished work.

She lives high up over the Vancouver harbor and keeps an eye on the comings and goings of freighters and tugboats, and the vagaries of the sea, the sea, the sea . . .

LaVergne, TN USA
07 December 2010
207779LV00003B/190/P